The Cocon Guide: How to Stay Healthy, Lose Weight and Feel Good through Use of Coconut Oil

by R. Johnson

Disclaimer:

The information contained in this book is for general information purposes only. This book is sold with the understanding the author and/or publisher is not giving medical advice, nor should the information contained in this book replace medical advice, nor is it intended to diagnose or treat any disease, illness or other medical condition. Always consult your medical practitioner before making any dietary changes or treating or attempting to treat any medical condition.

While we endeavor to keep the information up to date and correct, we make no representations or warranties of any kind, express or implied, about the completeness, accuracy, reliability, suitability or availability with respect to the book or the information, products, services, or related graphics contained book for any purpose. Any reliance you place on such information is therefore strictly at your own risk.

Dedication:

This book is dedicated to all those who have made the switch to coconut oil and all those who are thinking about making the switch. I switched over a few years ago and haven't looked back since.

Contents

What is Coconut Oil?

Coconut oil is an edible vegetable oil pressed from the meat of mature coconuts. The meat is ground down to a pulp and the oil is drawn out of it.

Pure virgin coconut oil is solid at room temperature in all but the warmest of climates. It begins to melt when it reaches a temperature of 76° F, eventually becoming a clear liquid. Cool it back down below the melting point and it eventually returns to a solid state.

Coconut oil in its solid state is sometimes mistakenly referred to as *coconut butter*. Coconut butter is similar to coconut oil, in that it contains the fatty acids of the coconut, but it also contains coconut meat and is a more buttery texture. Pure coconut oil only contains the fat. It doesn't have any coconut meat in it. The two are often used interchangeably in recipes, but there will be a difference in texture when the switch is made.

Coconut oil is made up of more than 90% saturated fat. While much has been made of the saturated fat in coconut oil, what isn't being said is the fats it contains have been shown to lower bad cholesterol and contribute to your health, as opposed to the fats found in many other vegetable oils, which have been shown to be bad for your health. Health organizations demonize saturated fat, and while there are saturated fats that aren't good for you, those fats aren't the type found in large amounts in coconut oil.

Coconut oil is an integral part of diets the world over. It's just now coming into its own in the Western world largely due to the unfair bad rap it's gotten, but it's gaining in leaps and bound as people realize the natural fats found in coconut oil are healthier fats than the ones they've been putting in their bodies.

In addition to being a part of a healthy diet, a vast array of benefits can be realized through external use of coconut oil. It can be used to boost the health of your skin and hair and is capable of treating all sorts of skin conditions, illnesses and ailments. Numerous studies have shown coconut oil to be beneficial to your health.

Stick around and learn what millions of people the world over already know. Coconut oil is largely innocent of the charges levied against it by health organizations in the Western world. It contains good fats that promote good health.

The Many Uses of Coconut Oil

Coconut oil is classified as a vegetable oil, but is used for a whole lot more than just cooking. Here are just some of the uses of coconut oil:

- **Cooking.** Coconut oil is a food staple in many cultures. It's the primary source of dietary fat in a number of cultures and is seeing rapid increases in popularity in Europe and the United States as more and more people realize the health benefits of this amazing oil.
- **Dietary supplement.** Coconut oil can be taken as a supplement to your diet. If you're cooking with it, this probably isn't necessary, as adding more coconut oil may add too much fat to your diet.
- **Apply it topically.** You can apply coconut oil to the skin by itself and it will melt right in. It can also be used as a massage or as a carrier oil that's combined with other oils.
- **Bath and body products.** From soaps to lotions, coconut oil can be used to make a number of healthy products that are good for you instead of being packed full of chemicals.
- **Skin and hair care.** It's good for both your skin and your hair. It regenerates and rejuvenates dry and damaged skin and protects your hair from protein loss and water damage.

- **Weight loss.** Watch the pounds melt away when you start using coconut oil. The fats in coconut oil are healthy fats that are easily processed by the body. Instead of being sent to the blood stream where they're converted to body fat, the fatty acids in coconut oil are sent straight to the liver, where they're used for energy.

Coconut oil is an integral part of many diets because it keeps the human body running like a well-oiled machine. All puns aside, avoiding coconut oil because of its saturated fat content means you're avoiding coconut oil because of one of its most beneficial constituents. Do the research and you'll find the mainstream health organizations are providing information about coconut oil that doesn't stand up under closer scrutiny.

The Health Benefits of Coconut Oil

Some people would have you believe coconut oil is a magic potion you can eat and rub on your body and watch as the extra pounds melt away and you magically become healthier and healthier. While I wholeheartedly believe coconut oil to be good stuff, I'm not going to try to sell you on the fact that coconut oil is a cure-all elixir like some of the literature out there tries to do.

Coconut oil has so many documented health benefits there's no reason to make stuff up. It's good stuff and can be a healthy part of most diets. Let's take a look at some of the key reasons you should consider adding coconut oil to your diet.

Medium-Chain Triglycerides (MCTs).

Medium-chain triglycerides (MCTs) are saturated fats, but they aren't like most other fats. MCTs are good for your body in a number of ways—and they comprise more than 2/3 of the total composition of coconut oil.

Other vegetable oils are largely made up of *long-chain triglycerides* (LCTs) which are nowhere near as good for you. They're more complex than the smaller MCTs and are harder for the body to digest and break down into energy. The human body has to use special enzymes to break LCTs down into a usable form.

The biggest difference between MCTs and other fats is the fact that MCTs aren't typically stored as body fat, while LCTs are. In fact, MCTs appear to enhance the body's ability to convert fat to energy and are a healthy source of energy for the body because they're sent straight to the liver. Studies have shown that calories from MCTs are used up at a faster rate than calories from LCTs.

Based on the fact that calories from MCTs are burned faster than calories from LCTs, it stands to reason that you should be able to lose weight if you switch from a diet high in LCTs to a diet that consumes the same number of calories, but is heavier in MCTs. You're taking the same amount of calories in, but will use them as energy at a faster rate.

Lauric Acid

Lauric acid is one of the many MCTs found in coconut oil. Also found in abundance in breast milk, lauric acid makes up nearly 50% of the total composition of coconut oil, making it one of the most abundant sources of lauric acid found in nature.

The human body changes lauric acid into *monolaurin*, which has antifungal, antiviral and antimicrobial properties. What this means is it seeks out fungus, microbes and bacteria in the body and breaks them down.

This makes coconut oil an effective natural remedy for bacterial infections, yeast infections and athlete's foot, amongst other things. It's also non-toxic, which is a definite strong point when you consider many of the medicines prescribed to treat infections and viruses are much harsher. Coconut oil is a powerful natural antibiotic that doesn't carry the same worry of building up resistance as man-made antibiotics because the body doesn't see it as an invader and start to build up immunities to it.

Monolaurin has proven effective in breaking down the following viruses:

- **Candida albicans.**
- **Flu.**
- **Giardia.**
- **Hepatitis C.**
- **Herpes.**
- **HIV.**
- **Measles.**

- **Pathogens.**

Coconut oil contains somewhere in the neighborhood of 6 to 8 grams of lauric acid in each tablespoon. There isn't a recommended daily intake amount for coconut oil, but some health experts recommend consuming 2 to 3 tablespoons per day.

Vitamin E Absorption

Don't be fooled by the literature out there claiming coconut oil is a good source of vitamin E. It isn't. A serving of coconut oil only contains 1% of the daily recommended intake of vitamin E. You'd have to eat 6 cups of coconut oil a day to get your recommend daily dosage of vitamin E from coconut alone.

What coconut oil does do is it helps your body readily absorb vitamin E when it is present.

In a 1999 study by the University of Western Ontario, coconut oil was determined to effectively promote absorption of vitamin E into the skin. While coconut oil in and of itself isn't a great source of vitamin E, you can use oil with vitamin E added to ensure your body is getting the vitamin E it needs.

Vitamin E is used by the body in multiple ways:

- **Aids muscle growth.**
- **Blocks polyunsaturated fats from oxidizing.**
- **Helps regenerate damaged tissue and heal wounds.**
- **It's an antioxidant that protects the body from *free radicals*, which are unstable molecules that can wreak havoc in the body.**
- **Moisturizes dry hair.**
- **Neurological health.**

There are coconut oils available that are already enriched with vitamin E or you can add vitamin E oil yourself. Vitamin E is commonly used in skin and hair care products because it moisturizes dry hair and regenerates damaged skin.

Naturally Healthy Skin and Hair

When was the last time you looked at the back of a beauty product bottle? If you haven't done it lately (or ever), you should stop what you're doing right now and read the ingredients on any one of the products on your bathroom counter. Most commercial skin and hair care products sold in stores today are packed full of harsh chemicals.

Sodium laureth sulfate and sodium lauryl sulfate are just two of the many poisons found in soaps, shampoos, toothpastes and any number of other products. They're in there solely to make your products foam up and make you think you're getting cleaner. Who knew that the refreshing lather you love from your favorite soap is more than likely caused by *surfactants* added to create that foamy feeling you associate with getting clean.

The reality is these chemicals may be doing more harm than good. These two chemicals alone can be responsible for damaging the hair and skin and can even cause liver toxicity as the liver attempts to process them. And rest assured these aren't the only chemicals found in your products. Most products sold over-the-counter today contain a cocktail of assorted chemicals.

Even the fragrances added to beauty products are potentially dangerous. Synthetic fragrances are cheaper and easier to use for aromatic purpose than natural oils and scents, so manufacturers often add man-made chemical blends to their products to provide scent. That honey lavender body scrub you're using may not have anything remotely close to honey or lavender in it.

Don't be fooled by products labeled as natural, organic or any number of misleading catch phrases designed to lure people into a false sense of comfort. When it comes to beauty products, these statements are largely unregulated. They definitely don't mean you're completely safe and are sometimes nothing more than a marketing ploy used to lure in unsuspecting buyers. The FDA doesn't usually step in until products are determined to be dangerous to your health. For new products on the market, that can take quite some time. For others, that never happens. A number of products on the market today contain suspected carcinogens—and nothing is being done about it.

Instead of making your skin and hair healthier, you end up masking the real issues while continuously pummeling your body with compounds it doesn't recognize and doesn't know how to process. This doesn't just place an unnecessary burden on your skin, it also places a heavy load on the organs tasked with processing these chemicals and getting rid of them once they invariably find their way into your bloodstream.

It's sad that people today are willing to sacrifice their health in the name of convenience, especially when there are natural products available that work with your body instead of working against it. Coconut oil is one such natural product. It can be used as a stand-alone product or it can be combined with essential oils and other natural products for an even bigger all-natural boost.

The nutrients found in coconut oil are good for both your skin and your hair. You wouldn't inject poisonous chemicals directly into your liver. Stop injecting them into your system by applying them to your skin and your scalp.

There's an entire chapter dedicated to using coconut oil for skin care later in the book. There's another chapter that discusses using it for hair care. Coconut oil gives you a safer alternative to the hazardous substances found in most commercial beauty products.

Still not convinced?

Read the label on the products you use and research the ingredients. I was literally disgusted when I found out for the first time what I'd been putting on my skin—and indirectly putting into my body. Stop pummeling your body with chemicals and start working with it.

Weight Loss

You'll often see coconut oil referred to as a natural weight loss supplement. You'll see other sources refuting this claim as untrue. I'll provide you with the scientific evidence and let you decide.

In a 2003 study published in the *International Journal of Obesity and Metabolic Disorders*, researchers from McGill University in Canada found that MCTs reduce stored fat in healthy overweight men. Another study completed by the same university in 2003 and published in the same journal concluded that consumption of MCTs in a targeted diet by healthy obese women "may prevent long-term weight gain."

When MCTs are compared to the LCTs found in oils commonly used for cooking, it becomes painfully obvious that they're a much healthier option. Calories from MCTs are used up faster by the body and aren't converted to body fat at the same rate LCTs are. You're much better off using coconut oil than you are oils that are packed full of LCTs like corn oil and olive oil. As long as you don't up the amount of calories you're taking in, it stands to reason that you'll burn the calories from coconut oil faster than the calories from the oils packed with LCTs.

This should, in theory, help promote weight loss.

One thing's for certain—it isn't going to hurt.

Switching to coconut oil alone probably isn't going to do you much good. Switching to coconut oil as part of a healthy lifestyle will work wonders. You'll start shedding pounds and will be able to keep them off because coconut oil doesn't turn into body fat at the same rate most other oils do. Since MCTs aren't passed through the bloodstream in the same way LCTs are, MCTs aren't stored all over the body as fat cells. Instead, they're sent to the liver where they're converted to energy. The body uses MCTs more efficiently than it does LCTs. Replacing other vegetable oils in your diet with MCT-heavy coconut oil replaces bad fat with good and boosts your metabolism.

Coconut oil alone probably isn't going to make a huge difference. Switching to coconut oil as part of a healthy diet will. Make the switch today and watch as your waistline vanishes.

Healthy Energy

The fats found in coconut oil are easily processed into energy by the liver. They digest quickly and are already broken down into fatty acids by the time they enter your intestines. Since they're ready to go and need no further processing, the fatty acids are sent directly to the liver via a vein called the portal vein without having to enter your circulatory system and travel through the rest of your body. They get to your liver faster and are easily broken down once they get there.

What this means is consuming coconut oil gives you a quick energy boost because the fatty acids are readily absorbed and processed by your body. This stands in stark contrast to the long-chain fatty acids found in unhealthy cooking oils, which go through a lengthy digestion process and are largely forced to circulate throughout the body via the bloodstream, where many of them are stored as fat long before they make it to the liver to be processed.

Consuming coconut oil can help cure fatigue by giving your body a quick energy boost to help you make it through the day. Take a teaspoon when you're feeling run down or add a teaspoon or two to a smoothie and you'll find you have energy reserves when you need them most. While the fats in other oils can leave you feeling lethargic and run down, coconut oil has the opposite effect.

Add coconut oil to your diet and you'll be ready for anything that comes your way.

Cholesterol Control

The first thing many people assume when they hear coconut oil is full of saturated fats is that it will raise cholesterol levels in the blood. This is true, but the cholesterol it raises is HDL cholesterol, which is widely considered by health experts to be good cholesterol. It lowers LDL cholesterol levels, which are considered to be the bad type of cholesterol.

A study completed in 2009 by the Universidade Federal de Alagoas in Brazil tested cholesterol levels in two groups of women, one group taking coconut oil and the other taking soybean oil. The group taking soybean oil saw an increase in overall cholesterol and the good HDL cholesterol level in their blood decreased. The group taking coconut oil saw increases in their HDL cholesterol levels and a decrease in the ratio of bad to good cholesterol.

While more studies need to be done, this indicates that coconut oil may not deserve the bad rap it gets because it's full of saturated fat. All saturated fats aren't created equal and the fats in coconut oil appear to work well once they enter the human body.

Fight Colds and Flus

The fatty acids found in coconut oil have antiviral properties that help the body ward off colds and flus.

Coconut oil can be used to prevent colds from taking hold and it also works well to help alleviate the side effects and may shorten the duration of colds once you come down with them. Take coconut oil as a supplement or add it to a warm tea to alleviate clogged sinuses, breathing problems, sore throats and coughs.

To further clear up congestion, add a few drops of eucalyptus essential oil to your coconut oil and rub it on your chest. Don't take coconut oil to which you've added essential oils internally.

Yeast Infections

Candida albicans.

For some, the mere mention of this word sends a shiver down their spine.

More commonly known as a yeast infection, a *candida overgrowth* occurs when candida bacteria grow out of control in the body. This growth can take hold in the mouth, the genitals or the digestive tract and can eventually begin to impact systems across the entire body.

Some of the symptoms of candida overgrowth aren't items you'd normally associate with a yeast infection. Here are some of the symptoms people are known to suffer:

- **Aches and pains.**
- **Bacterial infections.**
- **Bad smells.**
- **Blurred vision.**
- **Brain fog.**
- **Burning.**
- **Coughs.**
- **Dizziness.**
- **Dry skin.**
- **Fatigue.**
- **Fungal infections.**
- **Headaches.**
- **Inability to focus.**
- **Itching.**
- **Memory issues.**
- **Mood swings.**

- **Sinus infections.**
- **Sugar cravings.**
- **Thrush.**
- **White coating on tongue.**

It's estimated that 40 to 50 million people across the United States alone are suffering candida overgrowth. It's tough to pin down a solid number because large numbers of people go undiagnosed, either because they're embarrassed to admit they have a problem or they have no clue the symptoms they're suffering are from candida overgrowth.

This leads to people trying to treat the symptoms of the overgrowth, as opposed to actually trying to cure the cause of the symptoms. It's like trying to put out a blazing inferno by throwing a bucket of water into a single burning room. You might put the fire out in one small area, but it's still going to keep growing everywhere else.

Even people who are properly diagnosed and know exactly what's causing the problems they're experiencing have a difficult time treating candida overgrowth. Modern medicine is largely ineffective and can cause new health problems to present themselves. At times, the side effects suffered because of the medication can be worse than the effects of the candida infection.

When treatment does work, it often only works for a short period of time, after which the candida comes back with a vengeance. This leads to the growth of variants of candida that are resistant to antibiotics and hard to kill through use of medicine.

So what can one do to take care of a candida overgrowth that's growing out of control?

Luckily, there's a natural alternative.

Coconut oil contains caprylic acid, which is a powerful antifungal compound able to kill off the candida albicans species of candida. This is the candida species that causes the most problems in the human body. In a 2007 study published in *The Journal of Medicinal Food*, researchers Nigeria found coconut oil to be effective in killing candida albicans and other candida species. It has proven effective as a natural treatment and can be used to take the battle straight to the problem, as opposed to waiting for symptoms to present themselves and trying to treat them.

You're going to want to take it slow at first when you start using coconut oil to treat a yeast infection. Any attempt to clear your body of candida should be done under the watchful eye of a medical professional. If the infection is severe, your body could be full of candida and the associated die-off could cause medical issues to crop up. As much as you want to get rid of this harmful fungal growth right away, you don't want all the candida dying off at once.

Slow and steady wins this race.

For best results, start off consuming a tablespoon of coconut oil a day. Take a tablespoon a day for a week and then move your dosage up to two tablespoon s. After another week, move up to three, which is the dosage recommended by most natural health practitioners. Stepping up to three tablespoons slowly may help you avoid a massive candida die-off, which can result in moderate to severe flu-like symptoms.

For candida outbreaks on the skin, you can apply coconut oil topically to the infected area. For best results, apply the coconut oil topically up to 3 times a day and take it internally to kill off the candida in your digestive system. This two-pronged approach attacks the situation from multiple angles and is usually too much for the candida to handle.

After the initial die-off, you can add in a probiotic supplement to further crowd out the candida in your gut. Probiotic supplements are packed full of healthy bacteria that crowd out unhealthy candida.

This natural approach to attacking candida overgrowth eliminates candida from the system without use of Western medicines that may kill candida, but have a number of harsh side effects associated with them. Those having difficulty with candida overgrowth may want to give coconut oil a shot.

The Various Types of Coconut Oil

Refined or unrefined? Virgin or extra-virgin? Bargain-bin or high-end? What is fractionated oil?

There's no doubt about it. Novices to the world of coconut oil have their work cut out for them when it comes to choosing the type of oil they buy. Let's take a closer look at some of the terms you may see on the label and what they mean to you.

All coconut oils are classified as either refined or unrefined.

R*efined oil* is oil that's been processed to remove the smell and to kill germs and bacteria. The oil is usually odorless and doesn't taste like coconut anymore. This is the most common type of coconut oil used for cooking today. It's also used in a number of bath and body products because it doesn't impart the scent of coconut to the finished product. Refined oils have a higher smoke point and are typically used by people to cook foods without imparting the taste or smell of coconut to them. They contain some of the MCTs of their unrefined counterparts, but aren't as good for you as unrefined oil.

You may come across refined coconut oil that's *hydrogenated* or *partially hydrogenated*. Steer clear of these oils because they contain harmful trans fats that are created during the hydrogenation process. You're making the switch to coconut oil to get healthier, not to bombard your body with another round of dangerous fat.

Unless the label specifically says an oil is unrefined, it's safe to assume it's of the refined nature. Don't assume that all refined oils are the same quality. The refining process can leave behind contaminants like lye or toxic solvents. Steer clear of bargain-bin oils that use harsh chemicals in the refining process and make sure you're getting oil that's been extracted using a safe extraction method. If you go with refined oil, you absolutely need to make sure the refining process isn't adding anything you don't want in your body. If the process used isn't on the label, you may be able to clear things up by calling the manufacturer.

Unrefined oils are also known as *virgin* or *pure oils*.

These oils keep all of the health benefits of coconut oil intact. The oil has a coconut scent and flavor. Some people like it, while others are irritated that everything they cook has a slight coconut taste. To be completely honest with you, I cook with this oil frequently and rarely notice the coconut taste or smell. Some brands have much stronger coconut scents and smells than others, so don't be afraid to shop around until you find one you like.

Some unrefined coconut oils are labeled as *virgin*, while others are labeled as *extra-virgin*. There are no standards that clearly define the meaning of virgin vs. extra-virgin. Labeling coconut oil as "extra-virgin" is more of a marketing ploy than anything and you may come across manufacturers who sell "extra-virgin" oil at a higher price. They may or may not have used techniques that purify the oil in ways the virgin oils don't.

Organic oils are more expensive, but you should go with them when you can afford them. No pesticides or chemicals are used to grow the coconuts organic oil is made from. You don't have to worry about trace amounts of chemicals contaminating your coconut oil. There isn't a noticeable difference in the taste, smell or nutritional value of organic oil. The sole benefit is knowing your oil is free of chemicals and pesticides that are often used on commercial coconut trees.

Yet another type of coconut oil you may run across is *fractionated oil*. This type of oil has had all of the long-chain fatty acids removed from it. This is the most stable coconut oil and will last the longest before it has to be used. It may be even better for you than virgin coconut oil, but hasn't been studied enough for that claim to be made.

Still not sure which coconut oil you want?

Here's a handy list that should help you make your decision:

- **Never buy partially- or fully-hydrogenated oils. They're full of trans fats and aren't good for you.**
- **Buy organic whenever possible, but don't let the fact that you can't afford organic coconut oil stop you from using it.** The main benefit to organic oil is that it won't have trace amounts of chemicals left over from the coconut farm.
- **If you're cooking something and the smell or taste of coconut is a huge concern, go with refined coconut oil.** Notice the use of the word "huge" right there. If you can tolerate the taste and smell of coconut, you're better off going with virgin oils.
- **If you're cooking and the smell and taste of coconut is desired or isn't a problem, go with**

virgin coconut oil. This oil is by far the healthiest choice amongst coconut oils.

- **If you're looking for a natural sweetener that will add a light, sweet taste to your foods, go with virgin coconut oil.**
- **Virgin coconut oil is the best choice for dietary supplementation.**
- **Health and beauty products typically use virgin coconut oil.**

The best coconut oil overall is organic virgin coconut oil. Not coincidentally, it's the most expensive. If you can afford it, buy it. If not, go with pure virgin oil whenever possible.

No matter what oil you choose, always read the label. Make sure you're getting pure oil with no additives or coloring added. You don't want anything unnecessary added to your coconut oil. The only time I can maybe see allowing an additive is buying oil that has vitamin E added to it. Even then, it's best to buy virgin oil and add your own vitamin E. That way, you have control over the entire process.

Coconut Oil Extraction Methods

Boiling water, pressure, heat, chemicals and centrifuges are all used as coconut oil extraction methods. If something can be done to separate oil from coconut meat, you'd better believe somebody, somewhere has tried it.

Hydraulic presses are sometimes used to press the oil from the meat.

Coconut meat is placed in the press and large pistons are leveraged to squeeze as much oil as possible out of it. Ghani presses use the traditional method of extraction, which involves crushing the meat to get to the oil. This is one of the cleaner methods of extraction because the oil that is pressed out is pure and doesn't need to be refined. It's also one of the slower methods, which means it's rarely used to produce commercially-sold coconut oil.

Boiling water is another relatively clean method of extracting coconut oil. The meat is removed from the coconut shell and tossed in a big vat of boiling water. The heat causes the meat to soften up and release the oil into the water. Coconut oil is lighter than water, so it floats to the top, where it is skimmed from the surface and saved.

The cleanest oils are probably the ones extracted using *centrifuges*, which are machines that spin the contents placed inside in at high speeds. The meat is cut into tiny pieces and placed in the centrifuge, which spins at a speed chosen to separate the coconut oil from the meat. Oil extracted using this method is clean and has a strong coconut scent and taste.

Steer clear of *solvent-* or *expeller-extracted oils*. These methods use chemical solvents to extract the oil and trace amounts of the solvents invariably make it through into the final product. One solvent that's commonly used is hexane, which is a flammable liquid created while refining crude oil. While the level of hexane that makes it through the refining process is relatively low, it's never a good idea to willingly put petroleum byproducts into your body.

Go with coconut oil derived from one of the other methods. Your body will thank you for it.

How to Make Coconut Oil at Home

Buying virgin coconut oil pressed using a safe method isn't cheap.

If you feel up to the challenge, you can save a few bucks by making your own coconut oil at home following these simple steps:

1. **Cut or break the coconut(s) you plan on getting the oil from open and drain the milk.**
2. **Remove the meat from the shell.** A chisel works well to remove stubborn chunks.
3. **Grate the coconut to reduce it to smaller pieces that will be easier to process in the next step.**
4. **Place the meat in a blender or food processor.** You're going to need a good blender to blend coconut meat because it's rather hard.
5. **Add 1 ½ cups of water for every cup of coconut meat you have.**
6. **Blend until you have what amounts to a coconut smoothie.** You want the water to be creamy with tiny bits of coconut.
7. **Filter the coconut oil through cheesecloth laid across a bowl.**
8. **Repeat the filtering process 2 more times.** Each time, squeeze as much of the liquid out of the coconut meat that's left in the cheesecloth.
9. **Place the coconut water in an airtight container and securely fasten the lid.**
10. **Store in a cool, dark place for a couple days.**

11. **Pour the oil into a milk carton and store in a room with a temperature between 75 and 80° F for 12 hours.**
12. **Move the carton into the fridge and wait for the oil on top to solidify.**
13. **Cut the top off of the carton and scrape out the oil.**

You now have pure unrefined coconut oil you can use for whatever purpose you'd like.

Storing Coconut Oil

Coconut oil is one of the more stable vegetable oils, so it isn't as prone to going rancid as other oils. Virgin coconut oil is less stable than refined oil, because it hasn't been treated with heat, but it's still slow to oxidize and will last you a long time if you take the appropriate precautions.

There are a few items you need to be aware of that will speed up the process of your oil breaking down and going rancid. Heat, oxygen and light are your main concerns when it comes to extending the life of your coconut oil. Exposing your oil to any one of these three items will accelerate its demise. Expose it to all three at the same time and you'll have rancid oil in no time at all.

The best place to store your coconut oil is anywhere cool and dark. Screw the lid down tight to keep oxygen out and you should be good to go. Coconut oil lasts a long time before it starts to go rancid. Coconut oil can last a year or longer when stored properly in an airtight container.

To be completely honest with you, I've seen it last for a long time when stored improperly.

My aunt, who refuses to listen to my advice regarding coconut oil, has a container of virgin coconut oil she keeps on the counter in her well-lit bathroom. She uses it infrequently on her hair, so a single container can sit there as a long as a year or more. She rarely screws the lid on tight and her house is stifling hot in the summer because she refused to turn on the AC. I've opened the container to smell her current container a few times, sure it's going to smell rancid, but it keeps proving me wrong. It smells every bit as good today as it did 6 months ago.

I don't recommend storing your coconut oil in this manner, especially if you plan on cooking with it. I just wanted to include that story to show you the longevity of coconut oil and how hard it is to ruin. Any other unrefined oil left out that long would have gone bad a long time ago.

Aromatherapy: Use of Coconut Oil as a Carrier Oil

WARNING:

Essential oils are the powerful essences of the plants they're derived from. Most people are able to use them safely, but there is a small percentage of the population who has allergic reactions when they come in contact with certain oils. Use essential oils at your own risk and proceed with caution.

Aromatherapy is the use of aromatic plant oils to promote psychological and physical well-being. *Essential oils* are the oils contained within a plant that carry the essence of the plant. They're made up of a number of compounds that work together to give plants and flowers their unique scent.

Essential oils differ from coconut oil in that they're the chemical compounds that give plants their smell, while coconut oil is made up of fats from the plant. For those that are wondering, there is no real commercially-sold coconut essential oil. Coconut oil is as close as it gets.

In addition to smelling good, many of the compounds in essential oils are good for you. Each plant has its own unique blend of aromatic compounds. Physical application of essential oils to the skin allow the compounds found in the oil to enter the bloodstream, where they're able to go to work, helping your body in a number of ways. There are a number of therapeutic benefits associated with essential oils. Aromatherapy practitioners use them to treat everything from athlete's foot to the common cold.

While the many applications of essential oils are beyond the scope of this book, it's important to point out the fact that coconut oil can be used to deliver essential oils to the body through the skin. Essential oils are extremely strong compounds and it's rarely a good idea to apply them to the skin at full strength because they can cause sensitization issues and dermal irritation. Severe reactions can result in a person being unable to come in contact with certain oils without an allergic reaction for the rest of their life.

Carrier oils are used to dilute essential oils before they're applied to the skin. Small amounts of essential oils are added to carrier oils, which are then used to carry the essential oil onto the skin to minimize the risk of irritation. While there's still some risk, the risk is lessened because the oils aren't being applied at full strength.

Virgin coconut oil is good carrier oil because it's absorbed readily into the skin and is able to carry the essential oil into the skin as it's absorbed. Make sure you only use pure coconut oil, as some oils may have harmful additives that can cause irritation. The idea behind aromatherapy is to use *natural* compounds. Using a carrier oil with chemical additives defeats the purpose.

Many of the recipes in the next chapter make use of coconut oil's ability to deliver essential oils into the body through the skin. If you're using any of these oils for the first time, be careful, as they are powerful and can cause problems if they aren't used correctly. Always test new blends on a small area of skin first and wait to see if there's a reaction.

If there is, discontinue use immediately.

Coconut Oil for Skin Care

WARNING:

Coconut oil is largely made up of natural fats and is safe for most people. There are some people who show sensitivity to coconut oil, so always test on a small, inconspicuous area before use.

Skin problems can hit you with a double whammy. Not only are they painful and/or itchy, they're more often than not visible for the world to see. Having problems with your skin can really kill your confidence and can cause problems in other areas of your life.

School, work, your love life. All can be negatively impacted by a bad enough skin problem. You'll walk around feeling like you stick out like a sore thumb—and your negative feelings about yourself will be reflected in your attitude and the way you carry yourself.

The skin is the human body's largest organ. It's also the most visible. You'd think we'd take better care of it than we do, but most people ignore their skin and hope for the best. Sure, most people take showers regularly and wash their skin, but they largely ignore what their body is telling them. Others bombard their skin with commercial skin care products that ultimately end up making minor problems worse or causing new issues to crop up.

Nobody asks for bad skin, but there are a lot of things that can go wrong. From dry skin to acne, psoriasis to eczema, coconut oil may be able to help. One thing's for certain—it's worth a shot. People the world over are using it to ease the effects of various skin problems and diseases.

Here are some of the diseases and skin problems coconut oil is thought to be a natural remedy for:

- **Acne.**
- **Chafed skin.**
- **Cracked skin.**
- **Dermatitis.**
- **Dry skin.**
- **Eczema.**
- **Flaky skin.**
- **Itchy skin.**
- **Microbes.**
- **Oily skin.**
- **Pathogens.**
- **Psoriasis.**
- **Razor burn.**
- **Skin infections.**
- **Wound healing.**
- **Wrinkles.**

Coconut oil can help you achieve the healthy-looking skin you've always wanted. It has the following beneficial properties that can help your skin:

- **Antibiotic.**
- **Antifungal.**
- **Antimicrobial.**

- **Antioxidant.**
- **Emollient.**
- **Fights aging and wrinkles.**
- **Full of nutrients.**
- **Moisturizing.**
- **Nourishing.**

Best of all, it's completely natural and can be blended other natural ingredients like other oils, butters and essential oils. To use it, all you have to do is rub a bit of coconut oil between your fingers and massage it into your skin a couple times a day. It will melt as you apply it and will absorb into your skin, where it'll start to moisturize and clear your skin of a number of common issues.

You may have heard coconut oil clogs your pores.

This may be true of refined coconut oils because the refinement process raises the melting point of the oil and it can solidify in your pores. With virgin coconut oil this usually isn't an issue because the oil melts at 74° F. Your skin temperature is higher than that, so the oil will melt into your skin and stay melted. It won't solidify and clog your pores.

If you're using virgin coconut oil and are still having problems with clogged pores, it may be because you have large pores that are more susceptible to getting clogging. Try exfoliating before applying coconut oil. Then, instead of rubbing the oil in and leaving it like you would a moisturizer, massage it into your skin for a couple minutes and then wash it off.

Use of coconut oil can help you battle the effects of aging on your skin.

Young skin is smooth and supple because of the presence of elastic connective tissues. As you age, these tissues begin to break down. Wrinkles form as the skin ages and starts to sag.

Coconut oil stops this process dead in its tracks because it contains antioxidants that fight off the free radicals that are largely responsible for the destruction of these elastic tissues. Those who use coconut oil on their skin tend to have healthier skin with less wrinkles. It may not get rid of the wrinkles you have, but it can play a role in keeping them from getting worse. It may also stop new wrinkles from forming.

Using Coconut Oil to Cleanse Your Skin

Applying oil to your skin to clean pores clogged with oil may sound counterintuitive. Those with oily skin probably can't fathom adding even more oil to their skin, even in the name of cleanliness. Bear with me for a moment before dismissing coconut oil outright without at least considering the benefits.

Oil is naturally produced by your skin, and in and of itself isn't the cause of your problems. A certain level of oil is required in order for your skin to thrive.

Commercial cleansing products for oily skin strip your skin of the oil it needs to function properly. Astringent lotions and creams are the worst offenders, because they dry out skin that's already struggling to maintain its natural balance. The human body senses the skin is dry and has had the oil pulled out of it and starts creating *more* oil in an attempt to re-lubricate the skin.

This creates a vicious cycle.

You feel that your skin is oily. You apply a commercial product that's for oily skin. It dries your skin up by removing the oil from it. Your body senses the skin is devoid of oil and starts producing even more oil. It's a battle you're never going to win, and your skin ends up being the loser as it gets drier and drier and the body produces more and more oil with each cycle.

This is where oil cleansing really comes into its own. With this process, you apply coconut oil (or a castor/olive oil blend, which is the traditional way to do it) to your dry skin and rub it in. Let it sit for a minute and cover your face with a steaming hot washcloth. The coconut oil melts into your skin when you rub it in and the steam from the washcloth pulls it back out, along with the impurities and oil that's clogging your pores.

Once you've washed your face using this method, you'll find your skin doesn't feel oily or too dry because the coconut oil *naturally* cleaned out the pores and didn't set off another cycle of oil production.

I like to follow up the pulling treatment with another dab of coconut oil that I massage into my skin and leave there. It leaves my skin feeling soft and supple and I don't get the tight, stretched feeling I used to get when using astringent products.

Pure virgin coconut oil is the only coconut oil you should use for this process. Coconut oils with additives or refined coconut oils can cause clogged pores and other issues.

One warning about oil cleansing.

This method works for a lot of people. There are testimonials everywhere you look from people who swear by the process. There are a select few people that this process doesn't work for, and there are some who say it actually made their skin worse. If you decide to try it, closely monitor your skin for new issues popping up and discontinue use if it gets worse.

Homemade Skin Care Products

WARNING:

While generally considered safe, some of the items used in the recipes in this chapter have been known to cause skin irritation or allergic reactions in some individuals. The recipes in this chapter are for informational purposes only. Use them at your own risk.

When it comes to skin care, coconut oil works well on its own. It works even better when blended with other natural ingredients to form natural skin care products. The recipes in this chapter are all easy to make and are a treat for your skin, as opposed to commercial skin care products that contain harsh chemicals that can damage the skin.

All of the recipes in this chapter assume use of pure virgin coconut oil.

Acne Mask

NOTE: Apply this mask 2 to 3 times a week for best results. Massage it into your skin and let it sit for 15 minutes before washing it away with a warm washcloth.

Ingredients:

¼ cup coconut oil
3 drops lavender essential oil
3 drops tea tree essential oil

Directions:

1. Melt coconut oil in a saucepan over low heat.
2. Remove from heat and stir in essential oils.
3. Let thicken while stirring.

Bug Repellent Cream

Ingredients:

½ cup coconut oil
¼ cup Shea butter
6 drops Cedarwood essential oil
10 drops citronella essential oil
5 drops eucalyptus essential oil
10 drops rosemary essential oil
5 drops tea tree essential oil

Directions:

1. Melt coconut oil and shea butter together over low heat. If you want a thicker cream, melt a couple teaspoons of beeswax and add it to the blend.
2. Remove from heat and place melted blend in a small bowl.
3. Stir in the essential oils.
4. Let cool.
5. Store at room temperature in an airtight container.

Citrus Body Wash

Ingredients:

½ cup coconut oil
½ bar natural castile soap
3 cups water
3 tablespoons organic honey
5 drops lemon or orange essential oil

Directions:

1. Use cheese grater to grate the castile soap.
2. Add water to a pot and bring to a rolling boil.
3. Place soap in water and stir until soap has dissolved.
4. Remove from heat and let cool until lukewarm.
5. Place 1 cup of the soap mixture in a container that can be sealed with an airtight lid.
6. Add 1 ½ cups of water to the container.
7. Add ½ cup of coconut oil and the honey and stir until blended.
8. Add essential oils and stir until blended.

Citrus Sugar Scrub

Ingredients:

¼ cup coconut oil
¼ cup jojoba oil
½ cup cane sugar
10 drops lemon essential oil
5 drops lime essential oil
5 drops bergamot essential oil'

Directions:

1. Place coconut oil and jojoba oil in a saucepan and melt over low heat.
2. Remove from heat and place in a glass bowl.
3. Stir in the essential oils.
4. Wait until it cools to stir the sugar in.
5. Store in an airtight container until you're ready to use it.

Cocoa Body Butter

Ingredients:

¼ cup coconut oil
1/8 cup almond oil
¼ cup Shea butter
½ cup cocoa butter

Directions:

1. Combine all ingredients in a saucepan and heat gently until the butters and oils melt.
2. Blend together.
3. Remove from heat and place in glass bowl.
4. Let cool in fridge for 45 minutes.
5. Use blender to beat until light and fluffy.
6. Let sit in fridge for another 20 minutes.
7. Store in an airtight container in a cool, dark area.

Coconut Coffee Body Scrub

Ingredients:

1 cup coconut oil
1 ½ cups brown sugar
2 cups coffee, ground
1 tablespoon vanilla extract

Directions:

1. Place coconut oil in saucepan and melt over low heat.
2. Remove from heat and place in a container.
3. Stir in the rest of the ingredients.
4. Store in an airtight container until you're ready to use it.

Coconut Cold Cream

Ingredients:

½ cup coconut oil
¼ cup cosmetic beeswax pellets
¾ cup extra virgin olive oil
3 tablespoons rose water
2 drops eucalyptus essential oil
2 drops tea tree essential oil

Directions:

1. Melt the beeswax pellets, coconut oil and olive oil in a saucepan over low heat.
2. Place in a glass bowl and add the rest of the ingredients.
3. Whisk the ingredients together before the cream cools or it will set up without the ingredients being properly mixed.
4. Continue whisking as it cools. It should slowly turn into a cream.

Coconut Exfoliating Scrub

Ingredients:

1 cup coconut oil
1 cup sea salt
2 tablespoons vitamin E oil
½ a lemon

Directions:

1. Grind the sea salt into a powder. A coffee grinder works well for this step.
2. Melt the coconut oil in a saucepan over low heat.
3. Pour into a blender.
4. Add the rest of the ingredients to the blender and pulse until all ingredients are thoroughly blended.

Deodorant

Ingredients:

¼ cup coconut oil
2 tablespoons beeswax
¼ cup corn starch
¼ cup baking soda
Essential oils, for scent

Directions:

1. Melt coconut oil over low heat.
2. Add beeswax and stir until blended.
3. Remove from heat and let cool until the blend starts to solidify.
4. Stir in the rest of the ingredients.
5. Add a few drops of your favorite essential oils to add scent to your deodorant.
6. Store this deodorant in a jar or you can put it in an old deodorant stick and use it like regular deodorant.
7. If you really want it to harden up, you can keep it in the fridge. You might get some strange looks from friends if they notice you've got your deodorant in the fridge.

Lovely Lavender Bath Melts

Ingredients:

¼ cup coconut oil
½ cup cocoa butter
2 teaspoons almond oil
20 drops of lavender essential oil

Directions:

1. Melt coconut oil, cocoa butter and almond oil together in a double broiler.
2. Stir the blend together and remove from heat.
3. Let cool for 1 minute and add lavender essential oil. Stir it in.
4. Pour blend into molds and place in the fridge to harden.
5. Toss one in the tub before you take a bath for a lovely blend of oils, butter and aroma.

Lovely Lip Balm

Ingredients:

1 tablespoon coconut oil
1 tablespoon cosmetic beeswax
1 tablespoon Shea butter
1 drop chamomile essential oil
6 lip balm containers

Directions:

1. Melt beeswax in saucepan over low heat.
2. Add coconut oil and Shea butter and stir until melted.
3. Remove from heat and stir in chamomile oil.
4. Fill an eye dropper with melted liquid and use it to fill each lip balm container with equal amounts of lip balm.
5. Let harden and place the cap on the container.

Moisturizing Coconut Avocado Skin Cream

NOTE: Apply to skin and leave on for 15 minutes. Wash off with warm washcloth.

Ingredients:

2 tablespoons coconut oil
1 tablespoon honey
5 drops avocado oil
4 drops carrot seed oil

Directions:

1. Whisk ingredients together until blended.
2. Store in an airtight container.

Natural Tooth Cleaning Paste

Ingredients:

3 tablespoons coconut oil
3 tablespoons baking soda
1 tablespoon Bentonite clay
½ teaspoon xylitol
½ tablespoon peppermint extract

Directions:

1. Place ingredients into blender and blend until smooth.
2. Add coconut oil and blend until you get the texture you prefer.
3. Store in an airtight container.

Coconut Oil for Hair Care

People are usually surprised to find out coconut oil is great for their hair. After all, it's oil and the last thing most people want is matted, oily hair. Well, I've got news for you—coconut oil is every bit as good for your hair as it is for your skin.

In a study published in the Journal of Cosmetic Science in 2003, researchers found that coconut oil reduces protein loss in both undamaged and damaged hair when used both before and after washing the hair. When tested side-by-side with sunflower oil—another popular base oil for hair care products—coconut oil stood head and shoulders above its closest competitor. Surprisingly, sunflower oil did nothing to protect the hair from protein loss.

Coconut oil is a particularly effective pre-wash treatment for damaged hair.

When used before washing the hair, it naturally repels water from penetrating into damaged hair and causing further damage. Think of damaged hair as an old building that has a wood shingle roof. Some of the shingles are lifted, some are missing and some are cracked or broken. In a torrential downpour, water would find its way into the building, causing more damage. Now picture a layer of thick plastic being laid over the house. This would significantly reduce the amount of water getting in. This is what coconut oil does for your hair. It coats it and protects it from water making its way inside and causing more damage.

The fatty acids in coconut oil are attracted to the proteins in your hair and will make their way inside the hair shaft, essentially locking the proteins in. The more porous your hair is, the more you'll benefit from coconut oil. Those with naturally kinky or badly damaged hair may find coconut oil makes their hair more manageable and less prone to further damage.

Coconut oil can be used to reduce tangles in your hair. The added slip of the coconut oil reduces the friction found when dry strands of hair rub against one another. Instead of binding and knotting up, a strand of hair treated with coconut oil is more likely to slip and slide across other strands of hair, as opposed to catching on them and tangling. Adding coconut oil to already tangled hair may allow you more easily pull a comb or brush through the tangles.

Homemade Coconut Oil Hair Care Products

WARNING:

While generally considered safe for most applications, some of the items used in the recipes in this chapter have been known to cause skin irritation or allergic reactions in some individuals. The recipes in this chapter are for informational purposes only. Use them at your own risk.

You can use coconut oil as a prewash treatment, a post-wash treatment or you can rub it into your hair and use it as a conditioner that you leave in overnight. It works great on its own and will leave your hair looking lustrous and shiny.

Combining coconut oil with other natural ingredients allows you to further improve the health of your hair. Let's take a look at some of the recipes you can add to your ever-growing bag of coconut oil tricks.

Avocado Hair Softener

Ingredients:

2 tablespoons coconut oil
1 large egg
1 ripe avocado
2 tablespoons olive oil
½ cup water

Directions:

1. Blend ingredients together in a blender until smooth. There should be no chunks of avocado.
2. Apply the mixture to your hair and cover with a shower cap. Leave in for at least 30 minutes.
3. Wash your hair to get rid of all of the avocado.

Banana Coconut Dry Hair Conditioner

Ingredients:

2 tablespoons coconut oil
2 ripe bananas
2 tablespoons whole milk
1 tablespoon of raw honey

Directions:

1. You're going to need bananas that are so ripe they're starting to turn mushy. If you don't have bananas like this, let a couple bananas sit out until they ripen.
2. Add all ingredients to a blender and blend until smooth. Make sure there are no chunks of banana left.
3. Rub this conditioner into your hair and put on a plastic cap.
4. Let sit for an hour.
5. Wash your hair well. Make sure you get all of the banana out.

Brittle Hair Treatment

Ingredients:

2 tablespoons coconut oil
2 tablespoons jojoba oil
2 tablespoons olive oil
4 tablespoon mayonnaise
½ ripe banana

Directions:

1. Blend ingredients together in a blender until smooth. There should be no chunks of banana left.
2. Apply to your hair and cover with a shower cap. Leave in for at least 45 minutes.
3. Wash your hair thoroughly to get rid of all of the banana and mayo.

Coconut Egg Hair Conditioner

Ingredients:

½ cup coconut oil
1 egg
2 teaspoons raw honey

Directions:

1. Place the egg in a dish and beat it with a whisk.
2. Melt the coconut oil and add it to the egg dish.
3. Add the honey and whisk together until incorporated.
4. Apply this conditioner to your hair and scalp and massage it in.
5. Cover with a shower cap and leave it on for at least an hour. You can leave it in overnight if you'd like.
6. Remove shower cap and wash the coconut oil out of your hair with warm water.

Hair Spritz

Ingredients:

¼ cup coconut oil
5 drops lavender essential oil
5 drops geranium essential oil
Water
A spray bottle

Directions:

1. Add coconut oil to a spray bottle.
2. Pour warm water over the coconut oil. Fill the bottle to the top with warm water.
3. Once the coconut oil melts, add essential oils and shake until everything is blended.
4. When your hair needs a boost throughout the day, spritz it with this mixture.

Hair Strengthener

Ingredients:

2 tablespoons coconut oil
1 tablespoon almond oil

Directions:

1. Blend the coconut oil and almond oil.
2. Massage the blend into your hair and scalp.
3. Let sit for 30 minutes and wash it out.

Humble Honey Deep Conditioner

Ingredients:

¼ cup coconut oil

4 tablespoons raw honey

Directions:

1. Melt coconut oil and add honey.
2. Stir together.
3. Apply mixture to hair and let sit for 30 minutes.
4. Wash out of hair.

Natural Dandruff Treatment

Ingredients:

¼ cup coconut oil
¼ cup jojoba oil
10 drops tea tree essential oil
5 drops chamomile essential oil
5 drops patchouli essential oil
5 drops peppermint essential oil

Directions:

1. Stir essential oils into the coconut oil until blended.
2. Apply dandruff treatment to your head and massage it into your scalp.
3. Let it sit for 30 minutes.
4. Gently wash the treatment out of your hair.

Oily Hair Treatment

Ingredients:

2 tablespoons coconut oil
5 drops lavender essential oil
5 drops lemon essential oil
5 drops tea tree essential oil

Directions:

1. Blend essential oils into coconut oil.
2. Apply to hair and let sit for 30 minutes.
3. Wash from hair.

Scalp Treatment

Ingredients:

¼ cup coconut oil
2 tablespoons lemon juice
4 drops tea tree oil
3 drops rosemary oil

Directions:

1. Melt coconut oil and remove it from the heat.
2. Let sit for a minute. Add lemon juice and oils and stir in.
3. Apply mixture to your scalp. Be sure to really massage it in. Make sure you cover every inch of your scalp.
4. Cover your scalp with a shower cap and let sit for 15 minutes.
5. Wash out of your hair.

Cooking With Coconut Oil

An ever-growing group of coconut oil aficionados are using coconut oil as their main cooking oil. They love the fact that it can be used as a healthy replacement for butter and other unhealthy cooking oils.

They've grown to love and embrace the nutty coconut flavor this tasty oil imparts to their favorite dishes. While most cooking oils are heavily processed and are largely devoid of flavor, virgin coconut oil has a sweet coconut flavor that adds a bit of sweetness and a light coconut flavor to dishes it's used in.

Nutritional Information

The following nutrient data is for 1 tablespoon (13.6 grams) of coconut oil. It was pulled from the USDA National Nutrient Database for Standard Reference.

Item	Amount
Calories	117
Protein	0g
Carbohydrates	0g
Fiber	0g
Sugar	0g
Saturated Fat	11.76g
Monounsaturated Fat	0.79g
Polyunsaturated Fat	0.25g
Trans Fat	0g
Iron	0.01g
Vitamin E	0.01g
Vitamin K	0.1g

The first thing most health conscious people will notice is that coconut oil is made up almost entirely of saturated fat. Don't run away screaming just yet. The saturated fat in coconut oil isn't the same as the saturated fat found in butter and meat. This fat appears to help your body when consumed in moderate amounts, as opposed to harming it like other fats tend to do.

You probably also noticed the caloric load of coconut oil. While coconut oil does have a lot of calories, you're not going to be consuming much of it when cooking with it or using it as a supplement. A couple tablespoons a day is all you need to reap the benefits of coconut oil.

Even if you decide you don't want to *consume* coconut oil, there are other ways of reaping its health benefits. You can apply coconut oil topically without having to worry about the type of fat it has or how many calories it has in it.

What You Need to Know About Cooking Oils

Are you on a diet? Are you trying to lower your LDL cholesterol level? Are you looking for a healthy cooking oil that's gluten-free?

Coconut oil has you covered.

Replacing your regular cooking oil with coconut oil is a smart and healthy choice for most people. There are multiple reasons to make the switch. In order to understand why coconut oil stands head and shoulders above most other oils, let's take a look at the types of fats found in other oils.

Let's get one thing clear right away. All vegetable oils are not the same. Just because an oil is derived from a vegetable doesn't make it a healthy choice in the kitchen. In fact, a lot of the more common vegetable oils sold today like soybean, safflower and corn oil are heavily processed oils packed full of highly reactive fats called *polyunsaturated fats.*

These fats don't hold up well when exposed to high heat. They form free radicals under high heat, which can promote cell damage and degeneration, and they cause inflammation once inside the body, which is believed to be a contributing factor to diseases like heart disease and a number of other life-altering illnesses.

Even worse than polyunsaturated fats are trans fats, which are found in some oils. Trans fats have been tied to heart disease, diabetes, cancer, Alzheimer's disease and a number of other degenerative diseases. Hydrogenated and partially-hydrogenated oils are particularly bad, as they contain higher levels of trans fat than other oils do.

Canola oil contains trans fats because of the way it's processed. Researchers at the University of Florida at Gainesville found trans fat levels approaching 5 percent in some commercially sold canola oils.

In addition to popular cooking oils being sold with trans fats in them, there is also the worry of trans fat forming while you're cooking at high heat. While much has been made of this in various online forums and print publications, the truth is there probably isn't much to worry about when cooking at home. A 2012 study done by the National Food Research Institute in Japan found that trans fatty acids are indeed created when cooking in canola oil at high heat, but the level of these acids formed were fairly low after 10 frying cycles using the same oil. Unless you're reusing your vegetable oil over and over again at home, high heat probably isn't going to have much of an impact on the trans fat levels in your foods.

That said, it's better to not have to worry about trans fats forming in your cooking oil. Coconut oil is stable under high heat and is a good choice for cooking foods because of this stability.

Consuming Coconut Oil: All Saturated Fats Aren't Created Equal

Over the course of the last 30 years or so, people living in the Western world have had the fact that saturated fats are bad and should be avoided like the plague pounded into their heads. We've been told it clogs our arteries, contributes to heart disease and is largely responsible for a number of the health problems we're afflicted with as a nation. A number of health agencies have issued warnings against excessive consumption of coconut oil because of its high saturated fat content.

While coconut oil is indeed high in saturated fat, the majority of the fat found in coconut oil is good for you. The naturally occurring saturated fat in coconut oil is believed to actually improve the health of those who consume it. In order to understand why, let's take a step back and look at saturated fats as a whole. It's important to make the distinction between naturally-occurring saturated fats and man-made saturated fats.

Man-made saturated fats are fats that are processed into a saturated state through *hydrogenation*. This is a chemical process in which hydrogen gas is added to natural oils and a catalyst is used to force the oils to combine with the hydrogen atom. This process takes natural oils and coverts them into unnatural solids like margarine.

Most hydrogenated oils are only *partially-hydrogenated,* meaning the process is stopped before the fat or oil is fully hydrogenated. This process does nothing to improve the health value of the oils and creates a new type of fats that lie somewhere between saturated and unsaturated fats. These new fats are called *trans-fats.* You've probably heard of them and know how bad they are for you. They increase the level of bad LDL cholesterol in the body and negatively impact the good HDL cholesterol.

Hydrogenated oils and trans fats are used in the food industry in the creation of processed foods. They add structure and help the foods last longer and stick together better. If you're eating a lot of processed foods, you're more than likely consuming high levels of man-made trans fats, which are amongst the most destructive fats found in food.

So just how bad are they?

Your body gets no nutritional value from trans fats. Cancer, diabetes, heart disease, you name it. A number of ailments and diseases have been linked to consumption of these fats. To put it simply, the human body is not designed to handle hydrogenated oils. The more of this type of oil you bombard it with, the more likely you are to suffer health problems.

While coconut oil contains high levels of saturated fat, the fat in the oil is naturally occurring and is much better for you than hydrogenated oils and trans fats. In fact, there's ample evidence indicating the natural saturated fat in coconut oil is actually good for you.

Some tropical cultures consume coconuts as their primary form of dietary fat. If all saturated fats are created equal, one could surmise they'd have a high rate of heart failure and clogged arteries, amongst a myriad of other health problems. In a 1981 study titled " Cholesterol, coconuts, and diet on Polynesian atolls: a natural experiment: the Pukapuka and Tokelau island studies," researchers found that two populations of Polynesians with diets high in coconuts showed no evidence of harm from the higher levels of saturated fat they were consuming.

This isn't the only study backing coconut oil as being beneficial to your health.

Coconut oil contains a high level of lauric acid, which is a saturated fat known to increase good cholesterol in the body while decreasing bad cholesterol. In a 2004 study published in Clinical Biochemistry, researchers confirmed virgin coconut oil to be beneficial in lowering bad LDL cholesterol and raising good HDL cholesterol in lab animals. Yet another study released in 2009 concluded women who took 30 mL of coconut oil a day as a dietary supplement showed a decrease in abdominal fat when compared to women taking another kind of oil.

Much of the saturated fats found in coconut oil are medium-chain triglycerides (MCTs). Nearly 70% of coconut oil is composed of MCTs, which are easily processed into energy by the human body. These fats aren't believed to be as damaging to the body as other types of saturated fat. In fact, your body quickly processes MCTs and it's rare that they are stored as body fat. Contrast this with the long-chain triglycerides largely found in other oils, which are similar in form to the fat stored in the human body.

Moderate consumption of MCTs may promote weight loss and was shown to prevent long-term weight gain by boosting energy expenditure and fat oxidation in a 2003 study by the School of Dietetics and Human Nutrition at McGill University in Canada.

While there's undoubtedly a lot of research that still needs to be done on coconut oil, one thing's for certain. It's a great replacement for hydrogenated oils and partially hydrogenated oils and it's one of the healthiest vegetable oils around.

Baking with Coconut Oil

Coconut oil can be used to replace other fats in baked goods. It can usually be swapped out 1:1. If you have a recipe that calls for ½ cup of melted butter (or any cooking oil, for that matter), you can usually replace it with ½ cup of coconut oil. If you need melted coconut oil for your recipe, you can melt it in a saucepan over medium-low heat or you can fill the sink with hot water and place the container of coconut oil in the water for 10 minutes.

Try replacing the fats in your baked good with coconut oil.

You be surprised at how good it works. Leave your coconut oil solid and blend it into baked goods recipes that you want to be light and flaky. If you're using it to replace vegetable oil or melted butter, melt it and use it in its liquid form. Coconut oil is versatile enough that it can be used to replace unhealthy oils and shortening in most recipes.

If you're using cold ingredients straight out of the fridge like eggs and milk, you need to bring them to room temperature before adding liquid coconut oil to your recipe. Cold ingredients can cause liquid coconut butter to solidify in your batter or dough, which will result in small pieces of solid coconut oil floating around. If this happens, don't worry; you aren't going to have to throw out the batter. You can either blend it more to break up the chunks, or you can cook the batter as-is with the little pieces intact. I've had this happen a handful of times and it's never ruined the final product.

Sautéing and Deep Frying

The high smoke point for coconut oil makes it a good choice for sautéing and deep frying.

While deep fried foods aren't good for you regardless of what oil is used, coconut oil is one of the better oils to use for this task because it holds up well under high heat. You don't get the same dangerous free radicals that you do from other vegetable oils.

You can use coconut oil to sauté vegetables like leafy greens, broccoli, squash and zucchini. If you use pure coconut oil, it will add a slightly sweet flavor to your vegetables and you won't have to use butter or any other fats.

Other Uses in the Kitchen

There are so many uses for coconut oil in the kitchen it can make your head spin.

Here are even more ideas for adding coconut oil to your diet:

- **Add it to sauces.**
- **Add it to soups.**
- **Blend it into smoothies.**
- **Combine it with vinegar, honey and olive oil to make a tasty salad dressing.**
- **Drizzle it over rice.**
- **Flavor your coffee with it.**
- **Melt it and drizzle it over vegetables that you're roasting.** This gives your veggies a delicious flavor and gives your meal a healthy boost.
- **Scramble or fry eggs with it.**
- **Spread it on toast.** Add a bit of cinnamon for added flavor and an even bigger health boost.
- **Use it to pop popcorn.** You can also drizzle it on top of popcorn instead of using melted butter.
- **Use it to season a baked potato.**
- **Use it to season mashed potatoes.**

Be creative.

I'm constantly hearing of new and interesting uses for coconut oil in the kitchen. Don't be afraid to experiment. The worst that can happen is you whip up a batch of something that doesn't taste very good and has to be thrown out. And who knows . . . You might come up with something that's absolutely delicious.

Coconut Oil Food Recipes

Eating healthy doesn't have to mean eating tasteless, bland foods. Adding coconut oil to your diet gives you a healthy fat you can use to make a number of your favorite dishes healthier while imparting an interesting and delicious flavor to them.

The recipes in this section are some of my favorite coconut oil recipes. Keep in mind this is just the tip of the iceberg when it comes to using coconut oil in the kitchen. You can use it to replace other oils, butters and shortening in most recipes.

These recipes all assume you're using virgin or extra-virgin coconut oil. I suppose you could use refined coconut oil in most of them if you had to, but I recommend virgin oil because it's better for you.

Some of the recipes in this chapter call for white flour and refined sugars.

If you're on a gluten-free diet, swap the flour out with a gluten-free flour blend or switch over to almond flour. Don't switch to coconut flour because you can't swap your recipe out 1 to 1 from white flour to coconut flour. Coconut flour is extremely dry and will suck up moisture, so you have to add extra eggs, milk and other liquids to account for the desiccant nature of the coconut flour.

If you're trying to stay away from refined sugars, try switching over to agave nectar or honey. You'll have to experiment to get the flavor just right, but it's worth it when the result is a healthy treat that's both delicious and good for you.

Banana Blueberry Smoothie

Ingredients:

3 tablespoons coconut oil
1 ripe banana
1 cup orange juice
½ cup blueberries
1 tablespoon vanilla extract
Honey, to taste
5 ice cubes

Directions:

1. Add ingredients to blender and blend until smooth.
2. Add honey if you want the smoothie to be sweeter.
3. Serve immediately after blending.

Banana Oatmeal Smoothie

Ingredients:

3 tablespoons coconut oil
1 cup milk
2 ripe bananas
½ cup oats
½ cup almond butter
1 ½ teaspoons vanilla extract
2 tablespoons honey
5 ice cubes

Directions:

1. Add ingredients to blender and blend until smooth.
2. Add honey if you want the smoothie to be sweeter.
3. Serve immediately after blending.

Coconut Milk Eggnog

Ingredients:

2 tablespoons coconut oil

2 cups coconut milk

4 egg yolks

¼ cup honey

1 teaspoon vanilla extract

1 teaspoon ground nutmeg

Directions:

1. Blend all ingredients except nutmeg in a blender until smooth.
2. Pour into serving glasses.
3. Sprinkle nutmeg on top and serve cold.

Scrambled Eggs

Ingredients:

3 tablespoons coconut oil
3 eggs
3 tablespoons almond milk
Salt and pepper, to taste

Directions:

1. Place 1 tablespoon coconut oil in skillet over medium heat.
2. Melt coconut oil.
3. Tilt skillet back and forth to spread the melted oil across the skillet.
4. Add the rest of the ingredients to a bowl and whisk together.
5. Pour mixture into the skillet and cook, stirring frequently to ensure eggs remain scrambled.
6. Remove from heat and serve warm.

Easy Coconut Oil Waffles

Ingredients:

1 cup coconut oil
4 large eggs
3 cups milk
4 cups Cheerios, ground to a dust
2 tablespoons honey
1 ½ tablespoons baking powder
½ tablespoon sea salt

Directions:

1. Whisk eggs until frothy.
2. Whisk in the rest of the ingredients.
3. Pour batter into warm waffle iron and cook according to manufacturer instructions.
4. Top and serve warm.

All-Natural Homemade Granola

Ingredients:

2 cups coconut oil
1 cup clover honey
2 teaspoons vanilla
3 teaspoons cinnamon
6 cups oats
1 cup raisins
1 cup dried cranberries
1 cup sliced almond halves
½ cup shelled sunflower seeds, unsalted
½ cup shelled pumpkin seeds, unsalted
¼ cup flaxseed

Directions:

1. Preheat oven to 300 degrees F.
2. Melt coconut oil and honey together in a saucepan.
3. Stir in the vanilla.
4. Place all dry ingredients in a large bowl and mix thoroughly.
5. Add honey and coconut oil blend to the bowl and stir until everything is coated.
6. Grease baking sheet with coconut oil and place a single layer of granola on the sheet.
7. Bake for 50 to 60 minutes, or until granola starts to brown.
8. Set the granola out to dry.
9. Store in the fridge until you're ready to eat it.

Gluten-Free Bacon Breakfast Muffins

Ingredients:

2 tablespoons coconut oil
4 tablespoons coconut flour
7 strips bacon, fried and crumbled
4 eggs
½ teaspoon baking powder
½ cup cheddar cheese

Directions:

1. Preheat oven to 375 degrees F.
2. Add all ingredients to mixing bowl and mix until incorporated.
3. Grease muffin tin with coconut oil and fill each spot in tin with batter.
4. Bake for 15 to 20 minutes or until done.

Chocolate Cupcakes

Ingredients:

¾ cup coconut oil
2 eggs
1 ½ cups almond milk
1 cup water
2 teaspoons vanilla extract
2 cups sugar
2 cups flour
1 cup unsweetened cocoa
2 teaspoons baking soda
½ teaspoon baking powder
1 teaspoon salt

Directions:

1. Preheat oven to 350 degrees F.
2. Sift dry ingredients into a large mixing bowl.
3. Add wet ingredients and beat until blended.
4. Line a muffin tin with cupcake liners.
5. Fill liners ¾ of the way full with cupcake batter.
6. Bake for 20 to 25 minutes, or until a toothpick inserted into the center comes out clean.
7. Transfer cupcakes to wire rack and let cool.
8. Add topping or frosting and serve. These cupcakes work well with chocolate frosting with coconut sprinkled on top.

Coconut Chocolate Chip Cookies

Ingredients:

½ cup coconut oil, room temperature
2 eggs
2 cups oats
1 cup all-purpose flour
½ cup brown sugar
½ cup white sugar
1 teaspoon baking soda
½ teaspoon salt
2 teaspoons vanilla extract
1 cup semi-sweet chocolate chips
¼ cup shredded coconut

Directions:

1. Preheat oven to 350 degrees F.
2. Add coconut oil, brown sugar and white sugar to a mixing bowl and blend until smooth.
3. Add the rest of the ingredients and blend until incorporated.
4. Grease a cookie sheet with coconut oil and place 2-inch balls of dough on the sheet approximately 3 inches apart.
5. Bake for 10 to 12 minutes, or until cookies begin to brown.
6. Let cool for 10 minutes on cookie sheet.
7. Transfer to wire rack to finish cooling.

Rice Krispie Treats

Ingredients:

½ cup coconut oil
6 cups Rice Krispies cereal
4 cups marshmallows
1 teaspoon vanilla extract

Directions:

1. Add coconut oil and marshmallows to a saucepan and melt over medium heat.
2. Remove from heat and stir the rest of the ingredients in.
3. Pour mixture into a baking pan and press down until flat.
4. Place in fridge for 45 minutes, or until cool.
5. Cut into squares and serve.

Paper Bag Microwave Popcorn

Ingredients:

½ cup coconut oil, melted
2 cups popping corn
1 paper bag, for popping

Directions:

1. Place popping corn in paper bag.
2. Fold top over and place in microwave.
3. Let pop until popping slows down and there's only a pop every couple seconds.
4. Remove from microwave and place in a bowl.
5. Drizzle melted coconut oil over the top and enjoy!

Grilled Cheese Sandwich

Ingredients:

2 tablespoons coconut oil
3 slices of sharp cheddar cheese
2 slices of bread

Directions:

1. Distribute slices of cheese evenly between the two pieces of bread. Sandwich the cheese between the two slices.
2. Spread ½ tablespoon coconut oil on each side of the sandwich.
3. Place remaining coconut oil in a skillet over medium heat. Melt the coconut oil and tilt the skillet back and forth to distribute the melted oil across the skillet.
4. Place sandwich in skillet.
5. Let cook until first side starts to turn light brown.
6. Flip sandwich over and lightly brown the other side.
7. Continue cooking and flipping until the cheese is melted and the sandwich is browned to your liking.

Coconut Chicken Strips

Ingredients:

¼ cup coconut oil, for frying
2 eggs
1 pound chicken breast tenders, cut into strips
1 cup breadcrumbs
1 ½ teaspoons chili powder
½ teaspoon salt
¼ teaspoon onion powder
¼ teaspoon garlic powder

Directions:

1. Mix all ingredients except chicken, breadcrumbs and coconut oil in a bowl. Whisk until frothy.
2. Dip each chicken strip in the egg bath and roll it around in the breadcrumbs. Dip back into the egg bath.
3. Add coconut oil to skillet over medium-high heat and melt oil.
4. Place dipped chicken strips into oil and fry until golden brown on both sides.

Spicy Coconut Shrimp

Ingredients:

Coconut oil, for frying
12 – 15 shrimp, peeled and deveined
3 tablespoons lemon juice
1 tablespoon Cajun seasoning
½ teaspoon salt
½ teaspoon cayenne pepper

Directions:

1. Place shrimp in a plastic bag with seasoning and lemon juice and shake until well-coated.
2. Fry shrimp until they start to turn white. Make sure you cook both sides. This will take approximately 2 minutes per side.
3. Serve over rice or on a bed of lettuce.

Coconut Tilapia

Ingredients:

3 tablespoons coconut oil
1 lb tilapia filets
¼ cup coconut milk
2 cloves garlic, minced
½ cup coconut, shredded
2 teaspoons crushed red pepper
1 tablespoon lime juice
3 tablespoons fish sauce
1 green onion, diced
¼ teaspoon ground coriander
Cayenne pepper and salt, to taste
1 lime, sliced

Directions:

1. Make marinade by mixing coconut milk, 2 tablespoons of fish sauce and coriander.
2. Place fish filets in marinade. Coat both sides, place in fridge and let sit.
3. Brown coconut by placing in skillet on medium heat.
4. Stir until golden brown and remove from heat.
5. Place coconut in bowl with remaining ingredients and stir until incorporated.
6. Add cayenne pepper and salt, to taste.
7. Place 1 teaspoon of coconut oil in a skillet and melt over medium-high heat.

8. Place tilapia in pan and fry on one side for 90 seconds, then flip and fry for 90 seconds on the other side. Continue flipping and frying until fish is white and flaky on both sides.
9. Place fish on plate and top with coconut topping.
10. Squeeze fresh lime juice over the top and serve.

Sautéed Carrots and Onions

Ingredients:

3 tablespoons coconut oil
4 carrots, sliced into strips or coins
1 large onion, sliced into strips
1 teaspoon salt

Directions:

1. Place coconut oil in skillet and melt over medium-high heat.
2. Sauté carrots and onions until tender.
3. Add salt and serve warm.

Cheesy Mashed Cauliflower

I used to love mashed potatoes.

It was one of my guilty pleasures. I knew they were packed with starch and weren't really good for me, but I just couldn't give them up. That is, until I tried this mashed cauliflower recipe. I still whip up a batch of mashed potatoes over the holidays, but this is my go-to recipe when I'm craving something mashed.

Ingredients:

2 tablespoons coconut oil
½ cup grated cheddar cheese
½ cup cottage cheese
½ cup cream cheese
1 tablespoon garlic powder
½ teaspoon salt
½ teaspoon pepper

Directions:

1. Steam cauliflower until soft to the touch.
2. Place in food processor or blender and blend until the consistency of mashed potatoes.
3. Add the rest of the ingredients and blend until incorporated.
4. Top with more grated cheese or a drizzle of coconut oil. Serve warm.

Other Books You May Be Interested In

If you're interested in healthy eating, there are a number of other healthy foods you may be interested in adding to your diet. The following books may be of interest to you.

The Coconut Flour Cookbook: Delicious Gluten Free Coconut Flour Recipes

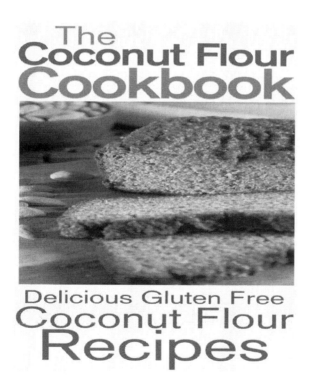

http://www.amazon.com/dp/B00CC0JFPM

The Almond Flour Cookbook: 30 Delicious and
Gluten Free Recipes

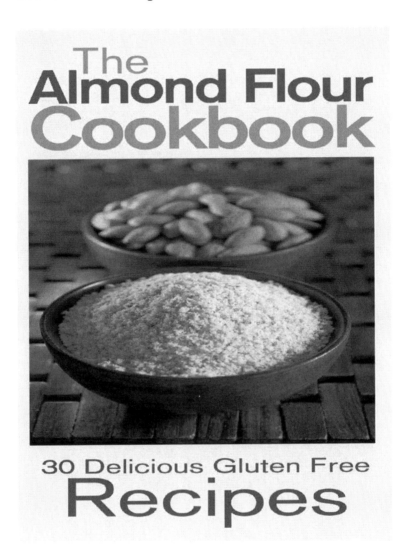

http://www.amazon.com/dp/B00CB3SJ0M

The Quinoa Cookbook: Healthy and Delicious Quinoa Recipes (Superfood Cookbooks)

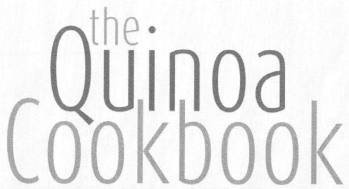

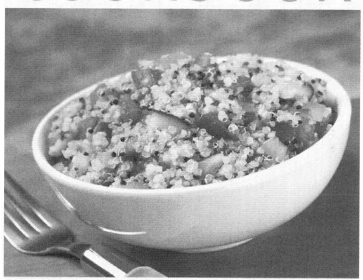

http://www.amazon.com/dp/B00B2T2420

If you want more information on essential oils and their applications, I recommend the following book:

The Aromatherapy & Essential Oils Handbook

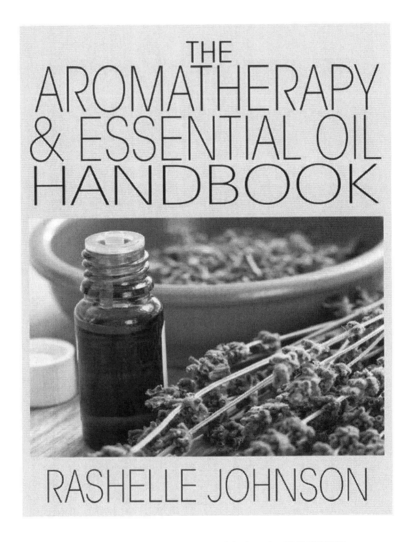

http://www.amazon.com/dp/B00BECCJXY

6023272R00063

Printed in Great Britain
by Amazon.co.uk, Ltd.,
Marston Gate.